The Essential Guide to Optimizing ADD/ADHD Treatment: Developing a Personalized Treatment Strategy

Austin Tallman

Questions may be directed to:
contact@TallmanPublications.com

Library of Congress Control Number: 2014917674

Paperback ISBN: 978-0-9897604-2-3
eBook ISBN: 978-0-9897604-3-0

Tallman Publications
PO Box 485
Spring Hill, TN 37174

If you need additional help learning how to perform the Excel operations detailed in this book, a DVD created by the author is available for purchase online. The DVD shows step by step how to do everything taught in the chapters that follow.

Visit: www.PersonalizedADHDTreatment.com for more information.

Table of Contents

Introduction

ADHD is a widespread condition affecting millions of Americans, both children and adults. This disorder takes many different forms and manifests itself in different ways among various individuals. With ADHD being so common, it's no surprise that there are countless solutions offered–everything from prescription drugs to behavioral therapy.

Unlike other publications that pertain to ADHD, this book does not promote any single treatment option. I am not claiming to have found some obscure miracle cure for ADHD that will make everyone better. Instead, this book does something different: it teaches you how to find the best treatment option for yourself or your child. According to my observations, ADHD frequently affects people differently. What works for one person, often times does not work for another. In our current health care system, doctors and other health practitioners who treat patients with ADHD simply do not have the time or resources to conduct an in-depth analysis for each patient.

Individuals who wish to effectively deal with ADHD must take an active role in the treatment process. One of the ways we can do this is by formulating our own system of research and working with our health care providers. By trying different treatment techniques, recording observations daily, and conducting simple statistical calculations on your computer, you can do a better job of discovering what works for you or your child–and what doesn't. This book will teach you how to conduct relatively complicated research in a way that is simple and easy to understand.

Note: I highly recommend that you use the computer program Microsoft Excel. While it is possible to utilize free online resources for the statistical work taught in this book, using Excel on your own computer will be much easier. This book will be instructing under the assumption that the reader is using Microsoft Excel for Windows PC.

Please note, this book is not intended to be a substitute for professional medical advice. Always consult with your doctor or healthcare provider before making any changes to your current health regimen.

Chapter 1
Introduction to the Idea

The Essential Guide to Optimizing ADD/ADHD Treatment is the result of an idea that occurred to me one day as I was pondering the inconsistencies in my own ADHD treatment. For more than a year, I had been intrigued by the fact that I was taking a constant dosage of prescription medication, yet still experienced good and bad days with my ADHD. Early on, I was able to make some observations about factors that had an impact on my ADHD and the effectiveness of my medication, but many things still lingered undiscovered. There were times when I was surprised because I would go through a day being able to focus better than expected, yet other days I could not focus despite having every reason to believe I would. I eventually surrendered to the idea that this was simply due to uncontrollable day-to-day fluctuations in body chemistry. However, while this may in part be true, I was wrong to believe that there was nothing more I could do.

Studying economics in college, I came across the use of statistics and something called regression analysis. We used regression analysis frequently in my economics and chemistry courses in order to determine how well a certain set of variables explained another set of variables. This tool was very useful for determining possible correlations between sets of data. So, what does this have to do with treating ADHD? After spending several months thinking I could never explain the daily fluctuations in my ability to focus, I put two and two together. Why not apply the same techniques used for economic analysis to the variables of my ADHD treatment? I devised a system whereby I recorded several aspects of my day, every day, and used statistics to help me understand how different things affect my inattentive-type ADHD.

Although this sounds overly technical and confusing, the truth is, this is a simple tool that is profoundly easy to interpret and understand. While it may seem daunting the first time you use this technique, it will be very easy to do once I walk you through the steps. Within this book, I will teach you how to employ these methods in order to better treat your or your child's ADHD. Due to the simplicity and incredible benefits of this system, I was sure that someone, somewhere, had written about this before. However, I was shocked when I was unable to find any published literature regarding the use of these statistical methods and ADHD treatment. For the first time, individuals and parents of children with ADHD have a way to conduct personalized research into the factors that influence a specific person's ADHD symptoms.

Chapter 2
Journaling

Formulating a System

The first step you must take when beginning your analysis of ADHD treatment is determining what factors you wish to study. Once you decide upon these factors, keep a daily journal of this information. This is open to anything you wish to include, which gives you the freedom to conduct a comprehensive analysis, but many people are unsure of where to start.

To begin, it's crucial that you find accurate ways of measuring ADHD symptoms. For adults, such as myself, who suffer from the more inattentive-type ADHD, useful things to measure might be daily focus, motivation, and productivity. I score these variables on a scale of zero to ten at the end of each day, but you may be able to find a more objective way to measure these factors depending on your particular circumstances. For example, if you work as a writer, you could record the number of words written/typed at the end of each day and use that as a measure of your productivity. Furthermore, as humans, we often succumb to bias when evaluating ourselves. If you spend a great deal of time with a friend or spouse on a daily basis, it may be helpful to find a way for them to evaluate your symptom control on your behalf.

For parents of a child with ADHD, there is an additional hurdle faced when trying to measure symptom relief. Your child may not be able to rank his or her ability to control their symptoms accurately on a daily basis. However, in cases where a child suffers from hyperactive ADHD, parents can often objectively rank their child's behavior daily. If your child suffers from inattention, and you believe this has a direct impact on his or her performance in school, finding a way to record grade averages may be a good way to measure treatment success over the long term. Try communicating with your child's teachers–perhaps they would be willing to rank your son or daughter's attention and behavior each day.

Once you have established how you plan to measure symptoms, you can begin selecting external variables that may be influencing those problems in either good or bad ways. As you will see in the upcoming examples, I personally like to begin by including any medications, vitamins, or supplements I currently take. It is a good idea to include practically everything taken since we are often unaware of things that may be impacting ADHD. Other good things to record include sleeping habits, physical activity, types of food eaten that day, and any side effects. Note any other factors that you believe may have an influence on treatment.

After putting together a list of variables to keep track of, you must then decide how you want to log the data. I made the decision to keep a record in file format on my computer using Microsoft Excel. This makes the most sense since the data will have to be on the computer in order to run the statistical analysis later on. One caveat though, is that it is important to regularly back up this file. You do not want a computer failure to result in the loss of all of your journaling work. For those who wish to work on paper, you can always keep a physical log of your information, but you will have to enter this into the program when you wish to analyze the data.

On the next page are two example logs with sample data shown in Microsoft Excel.

Date	Focus	Motivation	Productivity	Medication	Sleep (hrs)	Exercise (hrs)	Protein B-fast	Bread servings
1-Jan	10	10	10	1	8.5	1	1	0
2-Jan	4	3	4	0	5.5	0	1	3
3-Jan	6	7	7	0	8	1.5	1	0
4-Jan	8	6	5	1	7	0	0	2
5-Jan	8	10	9	1	7.5	2	1	0

Date	Focus	Motivation	Productivity	Medication	Ginkgo B (mg)	Magnesium (mg)	Egg B-fast	Insomnia	Headache
1-Jan	5	4	2	0	0	0	1	0	0
2-Jan	8	10	7	1	80	0	1	0	0
3-Jan	10	8	9	1	80	200	1	1	1
4-Jan	6	5	6	1	80	0	0	0	0
5-Jan	8	7	8	1	0	200	1	1	0

Putting Together a Log

The two samples on the previous page do not contain data from someone's actual ADHD symptom journal. However, they do present a good technique for putting together a log.

Across both examples, we study several external factors including medication, supplements, food, side effects, and lifestyle choices. Of particular interest are the numbers used to record each of these factors. When recording medication and supplement intake that may vary in dosage from day to day or over time, it is important to type in the actual dosage amount. If we record the intake of a supplement or drug without consideration for changes in dosage, this will lead to inaccurate, or less precise, results.

Since our goal is to find possible cause and effect relationships, we are able to include factors in our data that are not necessarily measured with numbers. For instance, in the first sample we observe whether the person ate a protein breakfast. In addition, we also record whether the individual suffered a headache. These are yes or no questions, so how do we include them? The standard practice is to assign the number (1) for yes, and (0) for no. Using these numbers is enough to establish a correlation between variables when conducting regression analysis.

The accuracy of your analysis is dependent upon your log. You may come across different factors that you can record with varying precision. For instance, in the first sample the log indicates whether the person suffered insomnia each day. In this particular example, the 1/0 (yes/no) designation is used. Keeping a record of it this way is fine if the person is generally awake for the same amount of time during each episode of insomnia. On the contrary, if the person is awake for differing amounts of time when they experience insomnia, it would be wise to ensure the log reflects this by recording time spent awake, etc.

I encourage you to take the time necessary to record detailed and accurate information. In the upcoming chapters, I will present additional information on methods for logging data.

Suggested Factors to Study

This section provides information on different factors that may be useful to study when managing ADHD. Please keep in mind, you should not consider this information to be professional medical advice. Your healthcare provider should ultimately handle treatment decisions. Always consult your doctor or clinician before making any changes to your health regimen.

Exercise

Many people report an improvement in ADHD symptoms when they exercise regularly. This should come as no surprise since physical activity is one of the best ways to maintain overall good health. Be sure to study the way exercise may influence your or your child's daily ADHD symptoms.

Food

In some cases, you may decide to keep track of variables that are specific to certain times of the day. This is particularly useful when trying to determine how different meals may affect ADHD symptoms, or how food impacts the efficacy of ADHD medication. In my personal experience, studying the impact various types of breakfast foods have on the functioning of my stimulant medication has been extremely valuable.

For myself and many others, eating eggs for breakfast has proven to be the most effective way to get the most out of stimulant medication. A full meal with any protein in general is good when taking medication after breakfast, and I have found that eggs, as the source of protein, seem to provide the best results. However, variations in the way the eggs are prepared may change the way the medicine works. Do you use butter, olive oil, or coconut oil? How about dairy milk or almond milk?

When I use butter to cook eggs for breakfast, I see a greater increase in my ability to focus and complete necessary tasks. In addition, using a small amount of almond milk in the egg mixture will precipitate a more calming, focused state when the medication begins to work. However, almond milk also predisposes me to a greater likelihood of getting a headache later in the day. Moreover, dairy milk has provided me with greater medication efficacy when consumed at breakfast whether in the egg mix or by itself.

These methods of food preparation may or may not affect you or your child the same way. Perhaps a different type of food altogether will provide you with greater benefits than eggs can. This is why we keep a log and test for correlations on an individual basis.

In addition to beneficial foods, there may be certain foods that have a negative impact on ADHD or contribute to symptoms similar to that of ADHD. For me, this includes breads, heavily processed foods, and chocolate. If possible, talk to your health care provider about testing for food sensitivities, as this may be a contributing factor for some people. It is also beneficial to keep a log that records focus, hyperactivity, etc., before and after meals of different food types. I have included an example in Chapter 4 that shows how to do this.

Nutritional/Herbal Supplements

This sub-section includes some of the most common nutritional and herbal agents used in the alternative treatment of ADHD. While all have been purported to have some possible benefit when used alone, some may also enhance the effectiveness of treatment with prescription medication. Although there are a limited number of scientific studies that provide information on the following supplements and ADHD, the techniques in this book will allow you to determine the efficacy of these supplements on a case-by-case basis. Always consult with your doctor before taking nutritional or herbal supplements, as many interact with certain medical conditions and prescription medications.

Vitamins, particularly the B vitamins and vitamin C, in many cases may help people with ADHD, according to published reports. I consume these daily as part of an overall health regimen. If you or your child takes medication for ADHD, be aware that vitamin C may inhibit many stimulant drugs if taken concurrently. To avoid this, I wait to take vitamin C until I am ready to go to sleep.

Fish oil has been touted as a helpful supplement for those with ADHD, although further research into its effectiveness is needed.[1] Fish oil can cause blood thinning in those who consume it, so be sure to inform your clinician that you are taking it. Avoid taking fish oil along with other blood thinning agents such as Ginkgo Biloba.

Magnesium levels in people with ADHD are often low. Some studies support the notion that supplementing magnesium may be beneficial, but further research is needed.[2] Many individuals claim that taking a magnesium supplement increases the effect of their stimulant ADHD medication and works to prevent or slow the process of developing a tolerance to that medication.

In my experience, small doses of magnesium have improved the effectiveness of my stimulant medication and have allowed me to remain on a lower dose than would otherwise be necessary. However, even doses of magnesium that are well below the recommended amount have caused headaches and insomnia for me on a regular basis when taken concurrently with medication. These side effects are reduced, but not entirely eliminated, when the supplement is taken late in the day, usually before going to sleep. I am not aware of these side effects occurring in the majority of people who take magnesium as an aid to their medication, although these side effects can occur in stimulant therapy alone. Most people who take magnesium supplements recommend against the standard form sold in most stores, magnesium oxide, due to its low rate of absorption. Instead, chelated magnesium or magnesium citrate is preferred.

Iron–People with ADHD frequently have low levels of iron in their blood, and some studies have linked low levels of iron in the brain to ADHD.[3] Upon investigating the use of iron in ADHD treatment, I discovered that I was, in fact, suffering from low iron levels that were barely above the threshold for normal. After adding an iron supplement, along with zinc, I noticed a slight improvement in my symptoms, both when I was taking stimulant medication and when I was not. However, there is uncertainty surrounding the potential benefit of taking iron supplements for ADHD, and it has been suggested that supplementation may not actually be able to change levels of iron in the brain.

Nevertheless, talk to your healthcare provider about blood tests to check iron levels, and discuss whether iron supplementation would be acceptable. **Never take iron supplements without consulting a doctor or other health practitioner first**. This is especially important for children. Too much iron can be fatal since the body does not have a major mechanism for releasing excess iron. Iron supplementation may also drastically change the way certain prescription medications function in your body.

Zinc–Like the other minerals mentioned thus far, some studies have suggested that individuals with ADHD sometimes suffer from low levels of zinc, and that zinc supplementation may be helpful in treating ADHD.[4] Consult your health care provider about whether or not you should add zinc to your nutritional regimen.

Ginkgo Biloba is an herb known for its ability to enhance cognitive function. It has been studied as a possible treatment for Alzheimer's, dementia, dyslexia and ADHD, among other things. One of the mechanisms by which this herb works is through increasing the chemicals in the brain necessary for focus.[5]

I have personally experienced positive, but mixed, results when taking Ginkgo Biloba alone. At high enough doses, Ginkgo has effectively reduced my tendency toward distraction, even when not taking any stimulant medication. However, it did not provide any motivational boost and was somewhat sedating. It also predisposed me to mild to moderate migraine headaches if I slept late on weekends, even though the herb is effective at preventing migraines for some people. Although my focus was greatly improved, I was not ultimately productive when taking Ginkgo Biloba as a standalone treatment.

Due to the effects of Ginkgo being an incomplete ADHD treatment in my case, I decided to try taking a small amount concurrently with my stimulant medication. The results of this treatment technique were highly favorable. Having developed a certain degree of tolerance to my medication over time, the Ginkgo Biloba proved effective at providing the necessary boost to my focus that I needed. In addition, the stimulant effect of my medication offset the drowsiness that frequently occurred while taking Ginkgo by itself, and the herb eliminated any insomnia that would have resulted from taking the medication. Many of the most focused and productive days during my senior year of college took place when I was taking stimulant medication and Ginkgo Biloba in tandem.

When taking Ginkgo Biloba supplements, the herb must build up in your system before you will realize any effects. Some report that they have to take the supplement for a few weeks before noticing any change. I generally sense it beginning to work the day after I first take it, and the effects peak after a few days of consumption. Like any supplement, in rare cases Ginkgo Biloba may cause problems. Ginkgo Biloba can cause blood thinning, so do not combine it with other medications or supplements that have the same effect. It is advisable to check with your doctor before taking it.

Ginseng is an herb known for providing increased mental and physical energy. It comes in several different types from various parts of the world. Some varieties of the herb have slightly differing functional characteristics compared to others. There are few studies that directly examine the use of Ginseng in people with ADHD, and much of the general research findings that involve the herb are contradictory. However, one study found that American Ginseng (Panax quinquefolius) did provide favorable results in ADHD patients when administered concurrently with Ginkgo Biloba.[6]

Conclusion

The takeaway message in this chapter is that external factors may affect many supplements and medications intended to function in a specific way, or they can work differently than expected altogether. Even if medication is the only path of ADHD treatment you choose to pursue, you may realize tremendous benefit in studying the variables that impact the way your medication works. Each person has unique body chemistry and things affect us all in different ways. The beauty of the technique taught in this book is that it takes these differences into consideration. Instead of prescribing a "one size fits all" solution, you will have the tools necessary to investigate and discover what works best for you or your child.

Chapter 3
Introduction to Excel

In this chapter, I will teach you how to perform the tests necessary to interpret the correlations within your journal data. Throughout this chapter, I will be using Microsoft Excel 2013 for Windows as my statistical software. However, the instructions should be relatively similar across different versions of Excel.

Before we begin the process of learning how to use Excel, let's go over a few basic things that are important to understand.

1. How much data do you need to perform an analysis? In most cases, the more the better. Throughout this chapter and the next, I will show samples that use 10 or so data entries, but you should be using much more. I suggest accumulating at least a month's worth of data before giving any credibility to your analysis. Once you reach 3 months or more, your data should be quite informative.

2. Remember to keep values/numbers in your journal in line with the other values recorded that day. If some numbers match up incorrectly with values from another day, your analysis will be completely off.

3. When displaying very small numbers, Excel will often reformat these numbers into something called exponential notation. For instance, the number 0.000001

will display as "1E-06." This is simply a way of expressing the number without displaying all of the zeros in front of the last digit. The "E-06" means that moving the decimal six places to the left gives you the full number.

4. Within this chapter and the next, I use the terms "dependent variable" and "independent variable" profusely. These are two statistical terms that are easy to understand.

Throughout this book, we will study the way independent variables affect the behavior of dependent variables. By "variable," we are referring to something that changes, such as the number of calories consumed day to day. Our statistical tests determine to what extent (if any) a dependent variable changes when an independent variable changes. One way of thinking about it is that the "independent" variable does what it wants, acting without any outside influence. We then try to see if the behavior of the "dependent" variable changes based on the behavior of the independent variable.

Frequently, we will test how medication (independent) affects focus (dependent). If you do not fully understand the nature of these terms yet, don't worry. As you proceed through the examples in this book, these terms will become second nature to you.

Now that we have some of the basic information out of the way, we are ready to begin using Microsoft Excel.

Making Sure Your Installation of Excel is Properly Set Up

The first step will be ensuring that you have the proper functionalities set up within Excel. Open a new worksheet in Excel and click the "DATA" tab at the top. Look for "Data Analysis" among the menu options within the data tab. It should be located in a subsection labeled "Analysis." If this is the first time you are using the Data Analysis feature within Excel, you might need to set it up.

If you are unable to locate the Data Analysis option, complete the following steps:

1. Click: File > Options.

2. When the Excel Options window has opened, select "Add-Ins" on the left-hand side.

3. At the bottom of the window, next to "Manage," select "Excel Add-Ins" from the dropdown menu. Then press "Go."

4. Under "Add-Ins available," you should see "Analysis Toolpak" and "Analysis Toolpak–VBA." Select both by clicking the checkbox to the left of each and then click "OK."

The Data Analysis feature should now be available for use under the Data tab.

Familiarizing Yourself with Regression Analysis in
Excel

We will be using something referred to as regression
analysis to conduct our research using Excel. Businesses
commonly use this statistical function to study
correlations between things such as the price and
number of sales for a particular product, but we will be
using it to determine what factors may be influencing
ADD or ADHD behavior. To begin, let's go through a
quick overview of how this tool works.

Within an Excel worksheet, I have entered two sample
lists of data. Notice that I have measured Focus on a
zero to ten scale, and Medication in milligrams.

Figure 3.1

	A	B
1	Focus	Medication (mg)
2	2	0
3	7	10
4	4	0
5	2	0
6	9	10
7	6	10
8	8	10
9	3	0
10	8	10

The "A" column contains the focus scores recorded on different days, and the "B" column shows the amount of medication taken on those days, if any, as measured in milligrams (mg).

In order to analyze this information, we must start the regression analysis function within Excel. We do this by selecting the "DATA" tab and then clicking the "Data Analysis" button that we enabled earlier. This brings up the following screen.

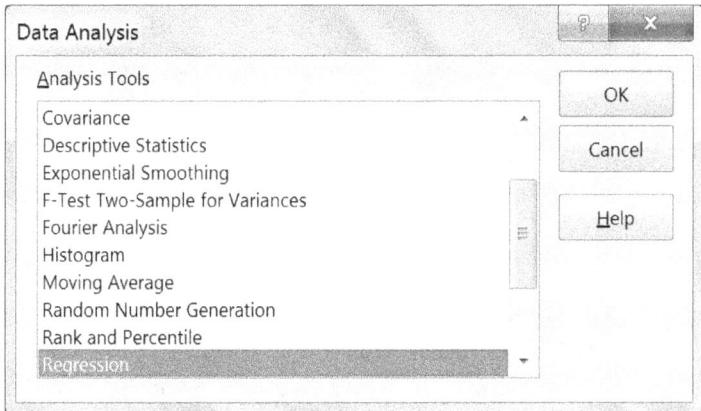

Scroll down until you find the "Regression" option, and select it. Then click "OK." The next window asks for the information we will be analyzing.

The **Input Y Range** contains the data referred to as the "dependent variable." It means that this is the information we are testing to see what influence, if any, the various factors of ADHD treatment have upon it. In this example, the Y data is the data within the Focus column (A). The **Input X Range** contains the data that is supposed to try and explain why the numbers in column A vary from day to day. This X data can be one column of information or multiple columns representing different factors of treatment. However, it should be noted that the Y data can only represent one column of information per test–in this case, focus levels from column A.

Using your logged information, fill in the requested data in this box as follows:

1. Click the empty **Input Y Range** box and then select the data in column A by left clicking the "Focus" box and moving the mouse down to the bottom of the column while holding down the mouse button. Release the mouse button. This will automatically enter the data into the Input Y Range box.

2. Using the same technique employed in step one, select the column(s) to be included as independent variables in the **Input X Range** box. In this example, this only includes column B with the values for Medication.

3. Select the box next to "Labels." This tells Excel that the first box in each selected column is not supposed to be a number, but rather a label for the data in that column.

The window with completed information should look something like the screen capture shown on the next page.

Press "OK" when finished. This will bring up the results of your regression analysis.

Figure 3.2

SUMMARY OUTPUT

Regression Statistics	
Multiple R	0.93165923
R Square	0.86798893
Adjusted R Square	0.84913021
Standard Error	1.06569897
Observations	9

ANOVA

	df	SS	MS	F	Significance F
Regression	1	52.27222222	52.27222	46.02586	0.000256863
Residual	7	7.95	1.135714		
Total	8	60.22222222			

	Coefficients	Standard Error	t Stat	P-value	Lower 95%	Upper 95%	Lower 95.0%	Upper 95.0%
Intercept	2.75	0.532849483	5.160932	0.001308	1.49001119	4.0099888	1.49001119	4.00998881
Medication (mg)	0.485	0.07148926	6.784236	0.000257	0.315954762	0.6540452	0.31595476	0.65404524

This may seem like an overwhelming amount of confusing information, but there are only a few things here that are relevant to what we are doing, and they are simple to understand. From here on out, I will not show the entire regression output that will appear on your screen as I have done on the previous page. Instead, I will only be including a condensed picture that shows the relevant information, such as the one below.

Figure 3.3

Regression Statistics	
R Square	0.86798893
Adjusted R Square	0.849130206
ANOVA	
	Significance F
Regression	0.000256863
	P-value
Medication (mg)	0.000256863

The explanation for each factor is as follows:

R Square: This number represents how well the independent variable(s) explain the dependent variable in percentage form. To understand this as a percentage, simply move the decimal over two spaces to the right. In this example, that gives us 86.8 percent (rounded). That means that 86.8 percent of the variation in focus each day in this sample can be attributed to whether or not the person studied took medication.

Adjusted R Square: When we include more than one independent variable (factors that may affect focus), it is important to ignore the R Square value and instead look at the Adjusted R Square. This is due to the fact that each time we add an independent variable to our analysis, the R Square value will increase–even if the extra independent variable does not correlate with the dependent variable whatsoever. The Adjusted R Square corrects this problem, and provides a more accurate measure of correlation.

Significance F: The number listed under Significance F is a statistical value that tells us how good our analysis (model) is. Typically, we want this number to be 0.05 or less. This value represents the probability that our correlation between the independent variable(s) and dependent variable occurred by chance. Obviously a smaller number is preferred because this indicates our data has greater credibility. If the Significance F value is 0.05, this means that there is a 5 percent chance that our correlation occurred by chance. In the case of our example, the Significance F value is 0.00026, indicating a 0.026 percent probability that our correlation is the result of pure luck.

P-value: The P-value tells us how significant a particular independent variable is within the model. If you are conducting an analysis with only one independent variable, as is the case in this example, then do not worry about the P-value for the lone independent variable. You will get all of the information you need from the other results. If you are running a regression with more than one independent variable, however, then you will want to check the P-value listed for each independent variable.

Similar to Significance F, the smaller the P-value the better. If there are independent variables included in your model with high P-values, you need to remove them. This is because the computer has determined that they are insignificant, and they are actually making it appear as if the variation of the dependent variable (Focus) is not as notable as it may actually be. Within the scientific research community, the usual standard is that a P-value needs to be less than 0.05 in order to be significant. A P-value of less than 0.01 is highly significant.

<u>Graphs and Non-Linear Data</u>

Regression analysis, as we have shown thus far, is useful for analyzing **linear** sets of data, but when the data is non-linear, we run into some problems. In this section of Chapter 3, I will show what makes data linear, and explain how non-linear data causes problems in our analysis.

Data is linear when one variable relates to another variable in an equal proportion. This results in a straight line when graphed. The graph on the next page demonstrates this using the following data.

Figure 3.4

Variable 1	Variable 2
0	0
1	1
2	2
3	3
4	4
5	5

Figure 3.5

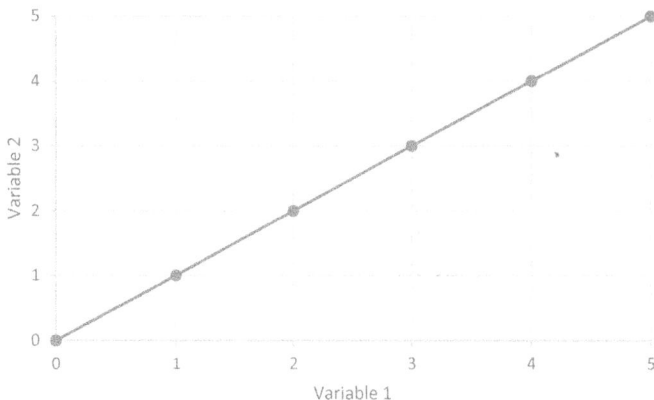

Since Variables 1 and 2 have the same numbers, we end up with a straight line when we place the values from each variable on a graph. Therefore, the two data sets have a linear relationship.

However, the numbers within two data sets do not have to be the same to be linear. Remember, on the previous page I stated that they must relate to each other proportionally. Therefore, if we have a data set with values that maintain a specific ratio, say 1 to 10, then there is a linear relationship. Take the following data for example.

Figure 3.6

Variable 3	Variable 4
0	0
1	10
2	20
3	30
4	40
5	50

Here we see that each time Variable 3 increases by one, Variable 4 increases by ten. Thus, they maintain a ratio of 1 to 10. This results in a linear relationship as shown by Figure 3.7 on the next page.

Figure 3.7

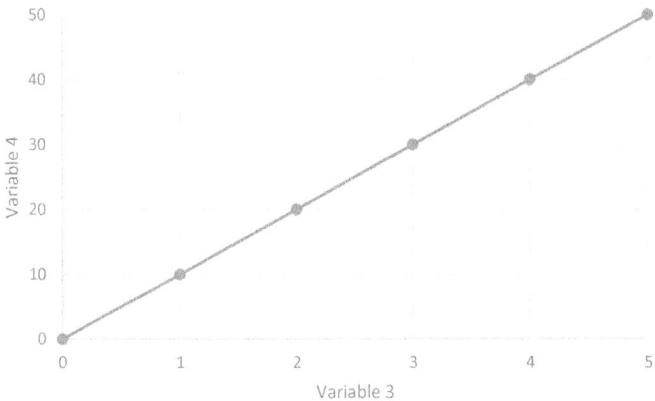

Linear relationships such as these are analyzed well using regression analysis. In fact, if you tried running a regression of these data sets, you would get a perfect R Square value of 1, simply because the relationship between the variables makes a perfectly straight line. However, in the real world things seldom relate to each other perfectly. Given this reality, we use regression analysis as a tool to determine how well things relate to one another. Take for example the following data that demonstrates a possible relationship between medication and focus.

Figure 3.8

Focus	Medication (mg)
3	0
2	0
4	0
7	10
5	10
7	10
8	15
9	15
8	15

A regression analysis of this data yields good results, with an R Square of 0.88 as well as P-value and Significance F values of well below 0.05. This signifies that there is a relationship between Medication and Focus; however, it does not represent a perfectly linear relationship. A graphical representation of the relationship is on the next page.

Figure 3.9

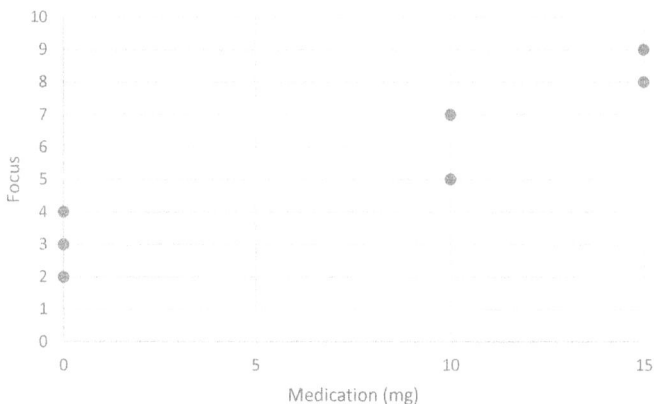

The large dots show where different values of
Medication and Focus correspond to each other based on
the data. Since these dots are not in a straight line, this
indicates that our variables do not have a perfectly linear
relationship. However, we are still able to discern
visually that as Medication increases, Focus tends to
increase as well. Even though our data points do not
create a straight line, we can still see that a relatively
linear relationship exists. I have added a "trendline" to
the chart to provide a better visual reference.

Figure 3.10

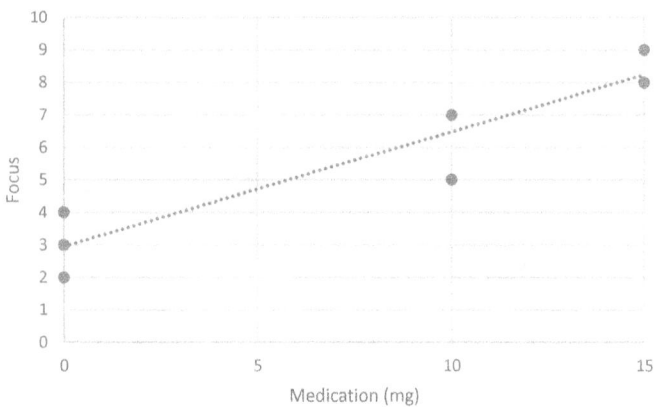

The trendline fitted to the graph shows the general relationship between the variables. This is what regression analysis does–it determines what line best fits the plotted data. If this was a perfectly linear relationship, all of the points would be on the trendline, and the R Square value would be one.

The linear relationships shown thus far are very compatible with regression analysis. However, when we try to examine data that does not have a relatively linear relationship, it can throw off our analysis completely. Take for example the data set in Figure 3.11.

Figure 3.11

Focus	Supplement (mg)
3	0
7	10
9	15
7	20
5	25
3	30

Graphing this data set gives the result below.

Figure 3.12

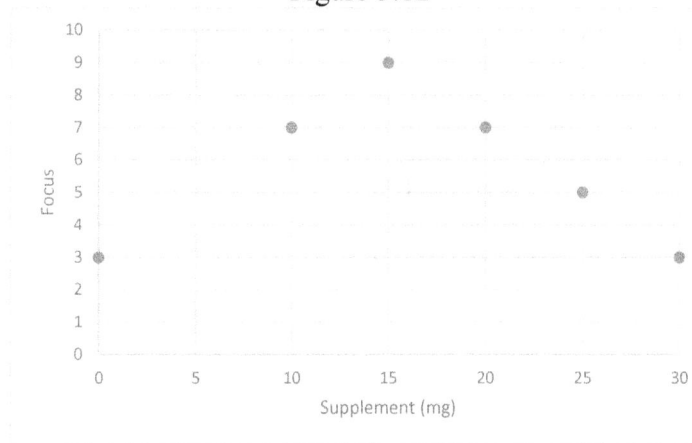

This is a good example of a non-linear relationship. As the dose of a certain supplement begins to increase, we notice a clear increase in focus. Once the supplement dose reaches 15 milligrams, any additional amount of the supplement causes a decrease in focus. Although there are countless reasons why we may observe a non-linear relationship, in this case we will assume that supplement doses of greater than 15mg lead to an increase in unwanted side effects, thereby lowering focus. Conducting a regression analysis of the data yields the following results.

Figure 3.13

Regression Statistics	
R Square	0.002597403
Adjusted R Square	-0.246753247
ANOVA	
	Significance F
Regression	0.923619109
	P-value
Supplement (mg)	0.923619109

The results of the regression suggest that it appears there is absolutely no correlation between the supplement and focus. The results are truly terrible. However, this makes sense because the computer is trying to determine how well the two variables relate to each other linearly. The dose of the supplement does explain the level of focus very well; however, the non-linear relationship ruins the ability of a standard regression to determine the correlation.

More advanced functions in Excel and mathematical techniques are available to run a regression of non-linear data. However, we will not cover them due to the nature and purpose of this book. Instead, I suggest that you determine the optimal dose, etc., that maximizes focus or whatever you are trying to increase, and only include data for that level going forward. In this case, we see that the supplement dose of 15mg results in the highest level of focus. Therefore, it would be best only to consume 15mg of the supplement and journal accordingly. Be sure to remove any focus data for supplement dosages different from 15mg, or it will hinder the abilities of the regression.

So far in this section, I have manually created graphs to show linear and non-linear relationships. You can easily do this as well by following these steps:

1. Start by selecting the two variables you wish to graph. Do this by left clicking and holding down the button while dragging the mouse from the top left corner of the data to the bottom right corner. This should create a thick green border around the two columns of data. By default, the variable in the left-hand column of the two selected is placed on the horizontal axis. I generally put the dependent variable in the leftmost column of my spreadsheet for simplicity, but this creates a confusing graph. If you have done the same, you will need to move your dependent variable data into a column to the right of the independent variable. This will ensure you create a graph that accurately depicts the relationship of the data.

2. Select the "INSERT" tab at the top.

3. In the "Charts" section, find the option for scatter charts. If you have trouble, running your mouse over each of the icons for the different charts will bring up a description. When you find the option for scatter charts, click it to show a drop-down list of chart options. Select the scatter chart in the top left portion of the box. Do not select a scatter plot with lines, as this may create confusing results.

It would be a good idea to create scatter plots for your data involving multiple dosage levels, at least in the beginning, in order to ascertain the linear/non-linear relationships of certain variables. It may also be helpful to create plots for data producing negative results that were not expected.

Further Information Regarding Multiple Regression

When we use several different independent variables to try to explain the activity of the dependent variable, we refer to this as "multiple regression." Multiple regression is interesting because it can be used to build a model over time that may accurately explain what influences ADHD behavior in a specific person. However, it requires some work to do it correctly.

Previously in this chapter, we surveyed the basic aspects of regression analysis using a simple data set that included one dependent and one independent variable. Now let's add another independent variable, making this a multiple regression.

Figure 3.14

Focus	Medication (mg)	Sunshine
2	0	1
7	10	0
4	0	1
2	0	0
9	10	1
6	10	0
8	10	1
3	0	0
8	10	1

Here I have added Sunshine as an additional independent variable. However, you'll notice that Sunshine is entirely random due to the fact that it perfectly alternates between yes and no (1 and 0). Let us observe how the addition of this variable changes the results of our model.

Regression Output of Original Model
Figure 3.15

Regression Statistics	
R Square	0.86798893
Adjusted R Square	0.849130206
ANOVA	
	Significance F
Regression	0.000256863
	P-value
Medication (mg)	0.000256863

Regression Output of Revised Model
Figure 3.16

Regression Statistics	
R Square	0.923012412
Adjusted R Square	0.897349883
ANOVA	
	Significance F
Regression	0.000456312
	P-value
Medication (mg)	0.000206822
Sunshine	0.083793998

You'll notice that the addition of the Sunshine variable caused the Adjusted R Square value to rise, but don't let this distract you. This variable is random and does not help explain why focus is varying day to day, yet it resulted in a clear increase in Adjusted R Square value. The Significance F value is also still well below a reasonable cutoff, indicating that the model is good, when in fact, it is not perfect. Looking now at the P-values, we notice that Sunshine has a P-value rounded to 0.084. This is greater than the 0.05 cutoff used in scientific research, indicating that it likely does not contribute to explaining the daily variation in focus. Therefore, we should remove Sunshine from the data.

Just for fun, let's see what would happen if we added another random variable. This time, we'll include a list of how many birds we see on each particular day. The data is as follows:

Figure 3.17

Focus	Medication (mg)	Sunshine	Birds
2	0	1	12
7	10	0	2
4	0	1	17
2	0	0	24
9	10	1	15
6	10	0	6
8	10	1	28
3	0	0	14
8	10	1	17

Regression output of third model
Figure 3.18

Regression Statistics	
R Square	0.925624038
Adjusted R Square	0.880998461
ANOVA	
	Significance F
Regression	0.002990492
	P-value
Medication (mg)	0.000784247
Sunshine	0.185169849
Birds	0.692600703

Here we see that the Adjusted R Square value is relatively unchanged, and the Significance F value is still well below a reasonable cutoff. Although we have considered the Significance F value "good" all along, we do observe it increasing with the addition of each useless independent variable, indicating that the overall model is decreasing in accuracy. Within the P-value column, we see that the P-value for the Birds independent variable is 0.69, which is incredibly large. Given this information, the amount of birds seen in a day clearly has no effect on focus, and we should remove it from the model.

It is very important to note:
The only reason that the Adjusted R Square and Significance F values remained desirable was because there was still one good independent variable– Medication. When we run the regression again without Medication, our positive results fall apart. Below is the regression output when Sunshine and Birds are the only independent variables.

Figure 3.19

Regression Statistics	
R Square	0.145710955
Adjusted R Square	-0.139052061

ANOVA	
	Significance F
Regression	0.623468494

	P-value
Sunshine	0.353923974
Birds	0.619175408

Chapter 4
Strategies and Analysis Examples

In this chapter, we will be going through examples to help solidify your understanding of regression analysis and charting as a tool to improve ADHD treatment. It is important that you read through each example in this chapter, even if some appear to be non-applicable to your situation. This chapter teaches broadly applicable analysis techniques through specific examples.

As a review from Chapter 3, below are the regression results we will be observing, as well as the values needed to establish possible correlations.

R Square: A value that gives the percentage of variation in the dependent variable explained by the independent variable(s). There is no commonly accepted "good" R Square value, but for our purposes it should be at least 0.5, and a value greater than 0.8 is likely to be a good indication.

Adjusted R Square: The value we look at instead of R Square when conducting a regression with more than one independent variable. We should see the Adjusted R Square value rise as we refine our independent variables and build a better model.

Significance F: This value tells us how well our overall analysis explains the variation in focus, hyperactivity, etc. Significance F values of less than 0.05 are generally considered acceptable.

P-value: The P-value tells us how significant a particular independent variable is in our model. An independent variable is considered an important part of our study if the P-value is less than 0.05.

Example #1
A Basic Case and the Nature of Positive/Negative Relationships

Similar to many of the examples shown thus far, this example studies the relationship between a single independent variable and our dependent variable. In this case, we will test the impact of a non-specific supplement on hyperactivity. We will chart hyperactivity in terms of how bad the symptoms are, with the number ten indicating the highest severity of symptoms.

Figure 4.1

Date	Hyperactivity	Supplement 1 (mg)
1-Jan	8	0
2-Jan	7	0
3-Jan	4	500
4-Jan	6	0
5-Jan	2	750
6-Jan	6	0
7-Jan	7	0
8-Jan	3	500
9-Jan	3	500
10-Jan	5	500
11-Jan	5	0
12-Jan	1	750

There are a few things to note from this data set. First, I have included a column of dates, which I assume you will do as well to maintain an organized data log. The date column should not be included when conducting a regression analysis or it will spoil the results.

Second, it is important to pay attention to the nature of the relationship between hyperactivity and supplementation. Previously, when using a measure such as Focus, we were looking at variables that may *increase* the Focus score. Now, with Hyperactivity, we are looking at variables that may *decrease* the Hyperactivity ranking. The ideal relationship between focus and medication is positive in the sense that increasing amounts of medication result in increased amounts of focus. Conversely, the ideal relationship between hyperactivity and a supplement is negative in the sense that increasing amounts of the supplement result in decreasing amounts of hyperactivity.

An alternative to this technique of charting would be to log the success of the management of hyperactivity instead of scoring the severity of symptoms. For instance, a score of 10 would mean that hyperactivity is being perfectly controlled, and thus the corresponding Hyperactivity Symptom Score would be 0. By instituting this change, you have made the relationship between the dependent and independent variables positive. This means that increasing amounts of the independent variable lead to increasing values of the dependent variable.

With all of this said, *it does not matter whether the relationship between your variables is positive or negative for the purposes of our analysis.* If we run two regressions, one using a Hyperactivity Management Score and another using a Hyperactivity Symptom Score, the resulting R Square, Significance F, and P-value will be the same in either case. This is because the correlation between the variables has not changed, only the positive or negative relation to one another.

TIP: If you have a column of data that you wish to change into a positive/negative relationship relative to another variable, see Appendix A at the end of this chapter for information on how to convert it automatically in Excel.

The analysis of the data shown in Figure 4.1 yields the regression results below.

Figure 4.2	
Regression Statistics	
R Square	0.819265144
Adjusted R Square	0.801191658
ANOVA	
	Significance F
Regression	5.15109E-05
	P-value
Supplement 1 (mg)	5.15109E-05

Figure 4.3

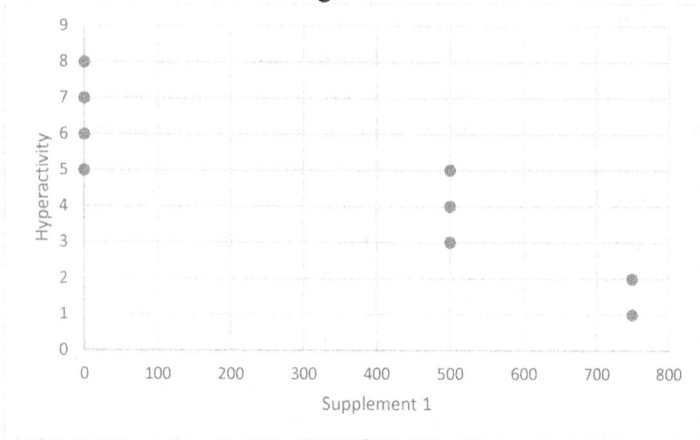

Since we used more than one dose of the supplement
during the data collection period (500mg and 750mg), I
have also included a scatter plot to do a general check on
the linearity of the relationship. A quick glance at the
plot shows that we are dealing with a relatively linear
relationship between Hyperactivity and Supplement 1.
**NOTE: Since the relationship between hyperactivity
and supplementation is negative, we expect to see a
downward sloping trend from left to right.** The group
of points at each of the three dosage levels charted for
Supplement 1 show the variation in Hyperactivity
observed at each dose of the supplement. The overall
trend between each dose level shows a linear, downward
sloping relationship as expected. Unlike the plot we
examined in Chapter 3, the points shown on this chart do
not create a "mountain" shape. Therefore, we need not
worry about deleting/altering data to fit our analysis.

At this point, there are only two values of interest we need to evaluate. Since this regression includes only one independent variable (Supplement 1), we examine the R Square value, which is 0.82. This is a decent value, indicating that 82 percent of the hyperactive behavior can be explained by the consumption of Supplement 1. To verify that these results are meaningful, we now turn to the Significance F value, which tells us the significance of our overall model. The Significance F value is 5.15109E-05, which represents 0.0000515109. Since the Significance F value is well under the 0.05 cutoff, we can conclude that Supplement 1 does have an impact on Hyperactivity. It stands to reason that it would be beneficial to continue taking Supplement 1 if it is medically advisable to do so.

Example #2
Refining a Multiple Regression Model

In this example, we will go through the process of building and refining a multiple regression model. Let's start with the following data set and regression results.

Figure 4.4

Focus	Med 1 (mg)	Supp 1 (mg)	Supp 2 (mg)
10	40	500	75
4	0	0	0
7	40	500	0
6	0	0	75
7	0	500	75
8	40	0	75
3	0	0	0
6	40	500	75
8	40	500	0
6	0	500	75
1	0	0	0
8	40	500	75

Figure 4.5

Regression Statistics	
R Square	0.732692539
Adjusted R Square	0.632452241

ANOVA	
	Significance F
Regression	0.011136165

	P-value
Med 1 (mg)	0.042721873
Supp 1 (mg)	0.296179246
Supp 2 (mg)	0.074987789

This analysis examines the effect of a medication and two supplements on focus. Unfortunately, our regression results are less than impressive. Our Adjusted R Square value is only 0.63, indicating that our model does not have a thorough grasp of the factors influencing Focus. Furthermore, the P-values for both supplements are above the 0.05 cutoff, suggesting that they are not useful predictors of Focus. In addition, the Medication P-value is below the cutoff, but not by much.

This exemplifies the need to include as many things as possible that may influence focus within our model. The medication and supplements in this example may in fact be tremendously beneficial for focus. However, if there are other factors with a major influence on focus that have not been included in the model, our results may be inaccurate and lead us to believe that medication and supplements are not as important as they actually are.

Let's add another independent variable to our model (Hours of Sleep), and see how the results change.

Figure 4.6

Focus	Med 1 (mg)	Supp 1 (mg)	Supp 2 (mg)	Sleep (Hours)
10	40	500	75	8
4	0	0	0	8.5
7	40	500	0	8
6	0	0	75	8.5
7	0	500	75	8
8	40	0	75	8
3	0	0	0	6.5
6	40	500	75	4
8	40	500	0	8.5
6	0	500	75	8
1	0	0	0	4
8	40	500	75	8.5

Figure 4.7

Regression Statistics	
R Square	0.946648857
Adjusted R Square	0.916162489

ANOVA	
	Significance F
Regression	0.00015129

	P-value
Med 1 (mg)	0.001533834
Supp 1 (mg)	0.10720753
Supp 2 (mg)	0.007692185
Sleep (Hours)	0.001125396

With the addition of Sleep to the model, our regression results drastically change for the better. Adjusted R Square is 0.91, and our Significance F value is well below the cutoff. Considering the drastic improvement in the overall model, and the P-value for Sleep being well below 0.05, it is apparent that sleep has been exerting a major influence over focus. In addition to the overall improvement, we notice that the P-values for the medication and supplements have dropped as well. In essence, this drop in P-values is because the regression no longer "blames" the medication and supplements for the previously unexplained variation in focus that was caused by differing amounts of sleep.

Although the model has improved, Supplement 1 has a P-value of 0.1, which is still above 0.05. Convention dictates that we remove Supplement 1 from the model, which yields the following regression results.

Figure 4.8

Regression Statistics	
R Square	0.920643017
Adjusted R Square	0.890884149
ANOVA	
	Significance F
Regression	9.4447E-05
	P-value
Med 1 (mg)	0.00035556
Supp 2 (mg)	0.00536901
Sleep (Hours)	0.001335069

Here we see that our Significance F value has dropped even further to an extremely small number, which is good. This indicates that the model is a strong predictor of focus, which of course means that we have successfully identified ways to improve focus. Our P-values have all dropped more as well since we have refined the model.

The takeaway interpretation from this analysis is that Medication 1, Supplement 2 and Sleep improve focus. Therefore, it would be a good idea to adhere to a treatment plan that includes those three–with the approval of a healthcare professional. Although we "technically" have removed Supplement 1 from the plan, I would still consider taking it. Its P-value of 0.1 excludes it from consideration as being "significant" by conventional standards, but it is still somewhat close. Although it may not be of major benefit, it may still provide a small amount of focus improvement.

Example #3
Testing for Side Effects

Although we have only used regression analysis to find ways to improve focus and hyperactivity so far, we can use the tool in countless other ways. In this example, we aren't going to try to find ways to improve ADHD treatment specifically. Instead, we'll use regression to determine if there is a correlation between headaches and our treatment.

Figure 4.9

Headache	Med 2	Supp 3	Supp 4
1	0	1	1
0	1	0	0
1	1	1	1
0	0	1	0
1	0	0	1
1	1	0	1
0	0	0	0
0	1	1	0
0	1	0	0
1	0	0	1
0	0	0	1
1	0	1	1

Figure 4.10

Regression Statistics	
R Square	0.746268657
Adjusted R Square	0.651119403

ANOVA

	Significance F
Regression	0.009103054

	P-value
Med 2	0.572602133
Supp 3	0.432830958
Supp 4	0.001609462

Looking over the log data in Figure 4.9, notice that all values entered are either one or zero. This is because we only recorded information as yes or no. As explained in Chapter 2, a "0" represents "no" and "1" represents "yes." Remember that when using this technique, yes or no must represent the same thing every time you use it for a given variable. In other words, "yes" must indicate the exact same dosage each time for Medication 2, otherwise there will be additional variation that the model will not discern. If dosages and headache severity vary, then you will need to use precise dose measurements and scores that indicate the severity of the headache.

Given these regression results, it would appear that Supplement 4 is likely the culprit causing headaches.

Our Significance F value is below the cutoff, suggesting that the regression has found something of interest. Furthermore, the P-value for Supplement 4 is well below 0.05, whereas the values for Medication 2 and Supplement 3 are nowhere close. Removing Medication 2 and Supplement 3 gives the following result.

Figure 4.11

Regression Statistics	
R Square	0.714285714
Adjusted R Square	0.685714286
ANOVA	
	Significance F
Regression	0.000537334
	P-value
Supp 4	0.000537334

Direct comparison further confirms our suspicion that there is a correlation between Supplement 4 and headaches. Significance F has become even smaller.

Example #4
An Advanced Analysis of Side Effects

This example presents a far more complicated problem
compared to what we faced in Example #3. As such, it
should help you develop the ability to analyze your data
in depth if the need arises. Take the following data and
regression.

Figure 4.12

Headache	Med 3 (mg)	Supp 5 (mg)	Supp 6 (mg)
0	0	0	0
0	40	0	0
0	0	400	0
0	0	0	50
2	40	0	0
0	40	0	0
0	40	0	50
5	40	200	0
9	40	400	0
8	40	400	0
2	40	0	0
0	40	0	50
0	0	400	0
0	0	400	50
8	40	400	50
1	0	200	0

Figure 4.13

Regression Statistics	
R Square	0.686868351
Adjusted R Square	0.608585439
ANOVA	
	Significance F
Regression	0.002363779
	P-value
Med 3 (mg)	0.002114254
Supp 5 (mg)	0.001454725
Supp 6 (mg)	0.705098232

In this example, we logged headaches on a 0-10 scale in terms of severity, and recorded the medication and supplements by the dose consumed. Looking over the regression results, it would appear that Medication 3 and Supplement 5 both clearly have a relationship with the occurrence of headaches. Supplement 6 does not seem to be relevant whatsoever, so it will be excluded from here on out.

Although Medication 3 and Supplement 5 both have P-values of well under 0.05, does this indicate with certainty that they both cause headaches? Not necessarily–there is the possibility that neither causes a headache by itself, but when taken together, a headache may result. If, in fact, a headache only occurs when we consume both Medication 3 and Supplement 5, then both will still show up as a cause of headaches in the regression. In order to discern what is actually going on here, it is necessary to break down the data and analyze it further.

To begin a more in-depth analysis, let's check to see if Medication 3 will cause a headache by itself. We want to do this by gathering all of the information we have about headaches and Medication 3 on days we did not consume Supplement 5. Referencing the original log data, we see that eight of the sixteen log entries do not include Supplement 5 usage. Figure 4.14 shows what data we will be extracting from the original information.

Figure 4.14

Headache	Med 3 (mg)	Supp 5 (mg)
0	0	0
0	40	0
0	0	400
0	0	0
2	40	0
0	40	0
0	40	0
5	40	200
9	40	400
8	40	400
2	40	0
0	40	0
0	0	400
0	0	400
8	40	400
1	0	200

Using the selected information, we can create the
following table of values.

Figure 4.15

Headache	Med 3 (mg)
0	0
0	40
0	0
2	40
0	40
0	40
2	40
0	40

By extracting the Headache and Medication 3 data when Supplement 5 is zero, we are isolating the behavior of Medication 3 from any possible influence/interaction with Supplement 5 that could be causing headaches. Running a regression with Headache as the dependent variable and Medication 3 as the independent variable gives the following result.

Figure 4.16

Regression Statistics	
R Square	0.111111111
Adjusted R Square	-0.037037037
ANOVA	
	Significance F
Regression	0.419753086
	P-value
Med 3 (mg)	0.419753086

Studying the relationship between the Headache variable and Medication 3 reveals that Medication 3 alone really has hardly any correlation with headaches. We know now that Medication 3 is only associated with headaches when Supplement 5 is taken at the same time. If you are satisfied with this information, then no further analysis is necessary. However, we can still discover more information regarding the nature of the cause of the headaches.

Now that we know headaches generally only occur during treatment with Medication 3 when taken concurrently with Supplement 5, let us check to see if Supplement 5 causes headaches by itself. We can do so by compiling all of the data we have on headaches and Supplement 5 when Medication 3 is not taken (zero). This results in the data in Figure 4.17 and the regression results that follow.

Figure 4.17

Headache	Supp 5 (mg)
0	0
0	400
0	0
0	400
0	400
1	200

Figure 4.18

Regression Statistics	
R Square	0.006896552
Adjusted R Square	-0.24137931

ANOVA

	Significance F
Regression	0.875718144

	P-value
Supp 5 (mg)	0.875718144

The regression analyzing the isolated behavior of Supplement 5 also reveals no significant correlation with headaches. Therefore, it is reasonable to conclude that neither Medication 3 nor Supplement 5 causes a headache on its own. Rather, the two interact when taken concurrently, resulting in a headache.

If you are interested in confirming this conclusion, then the analysis could be taken one step further. We can compile data to analyze in a specific way by simply proposing a question for the regression to answer: When taking Medication 3, does the consumption of Supplement 5 cause a headache? We prepare the information to answer that question by selecting the following data.

Figure 4.19

Headache	Med 3 (mg)	Supp 5 (mg)
0	0	0
0	40	0
0	0	400
0	0	0
2	40	0
0	40	0
0	40	0
5	40	200
9	40	400
8	40	400
2	40	0
0	40	0
0	0	400
0	0	400
8	40	400
1	0	200

Which is then compiled as follows on the next page.

Figure 4.20

Headache	Supp 5 (mg)
0	0
2	0
0	0
0	0
5	200
9	400
8	400
2	0
0	0
8	400

By putting together the Headache and Supplement 5 data only when Medication 3 is taken, we are able to test whether or not a headache occurs when they are taken together. The regression results are below.

Figure 4.21

Regression Statistics	
R Square	0.950773558
Adjusted R Square	0.944620253

ANOVA	
	Significance F
Regression	1.63828E-06

	P-value
Supp 5 (mg)	1.63828E-06

From this information, we can confirm that there is a strong correlation between headaches and the concurrent dosing of Medication 3 and Supplement 5.

NOTE: You'll notice in this last step that I tested whether or not the consumption of Supplement 5 makes a difference when Medication 3 is already being taken. This is because the dosage for Medication 3 is constant (40mg). If I had tested log data when both Medication 3 and Supplement 5 were fluctuating doses, this would have skewed the result. When doing this sort of test, you need to compare one independent variable that is fluctuating (even if it is just going between no dose and a constant dose) while the other independent variable remains constant against the dependent variable.

You can also use this same technique to test whether or not a particular supplement increases the efficacy of another supplement or medication. Although a supplement may not have a beneficial effect when taken alone, it could work in tandem with something else to improve treatment. Running these tests may reveal that some things which appear to be of little value, are actually significant in an indirect sense.

Example #5
Analyzing the Effect of Food and Multiple Time Periods

Up until now, we have only studied hyperactivity and focus using a score that represents the entire day. However, it is possible to break that down even further and investigate symptoms at different times of the day. For instance, how does focus change after consuming a meal?

Let's begin with the following table of data.

Figure 4.22

Focus prior	Focus after	Difference in Focus	Chicken	Vegetables	Bread	Medication
8	8	0	0	1	0	1
7	8	1	2	1	0	1
8	4	-4	0	0	2	1
7	5	-2	0	1	1	1
6	5	-1	1	1	0	1
9	4	-5	0	0	4	1
8	5	-3	1	1	2	1
7	6	-1	1	1	0	1

You'll notice that this table has two columns of Focus scores instead of just one. Focus is scored prior to the meal, and at a set time following the meal, such as 30 minutes or an hour afterward. In this case, it would be poor judgment to wait too long after the meal to evaluate focus, or we may start to see a decrease simply because the medication is wearing off. We calculate the difference between the Focus scores by subtracting the "prior" Focus from the "after" Focus. Excel can compute the difference automatically when you enter an equation such as "=B1-A1" and follow the steps detailed in Appendix A of this chapter. When there has been a decrease in focus following the meal, the "Difference in Focus" value is negative.

To the right of the columns containing focus data, there are three independent variables: Chicken, Vegetables and Bread. The first two independent variables are recorded using the yes/no, 1/0 system. It would be more accurate to log precise serving amounts, although this may be very difficult to do effectively. You might try using the 1/0 method of recording, and then, if an extremely large portion of say, chicken, is consumed, you score it at 2 in that instance.

We logged Medication in the column farthest to the right. However, Medication is not to be included in the regression. We need to observe the impact of food without external influences distorting the results. Given this requirement, we only include logged entries in the table that include the use of medication since we can assume that using (or not using) medication has a significant impact on focus. If a log entry was made when medication had not been consumed, it would need to be excluded from this table and our analysis. We include the column for Medication as a way of making sure we analyze food when the other influencing factors are constant. In this case, we are examining the effects of food while taking medication; however, you could also study the effects of food when you have not taken any medication.

Since we are trying to find a possible **change** in focus due to eating certain foods, we do not use Focus scores as our dependent variable. Instead, we use "Difference in Focus" as the dependent variable, since it measures any change in focus. The results of our regression are below.

Figure 4.23

Regression Statistics	
R Square	0.889328063
Adjusted R Square	0.806324111

ANOVA	
	Significance F
Regression	0.022099901

	P-value
Chicken	0.384930749
Vegetables	0.73207605
Bread	0.053215412

Examination of the Significance F indicates that our model has likely found something of interest. Looking down at the P-values, Chicken appears to be insignificant, and Vegetables even more so. The P-value for Bread is 0.053, which is technically just above the cutoff for significance. However, if Bread is in fact significant, its P-value is distorted by any non-significant variables in the model, such as Chicken and Vegetables. Since the Significance F value tells us we have something, and the Chicken and Vegetable variables are clearly irrelevant, let's run the regression again using only Bread as the independent variable.

Figure 4.24

Regression Statistics		
R Square	0.851576994	
Adjusted R Square	0.826839827	
ANOVA		
	Significance F	
Regression	0.001084294	
	Coefficients	P-value
Bread	-1.285714286	0.001084294

The revised regression shows a clear relationship between bread consumption and a decrease in focus. Although, how do we know for sure that the bread is decreasing focus instead of increasing it? An examination of the original data table shows that focus generally decreases when bread is consumed. However, manual examination is imprecise and cumbersome in larger data sets. A quick way to verify the nature of the established relationship is to check the "Coefficients" value for Bread. Since the coefficient is a negative value (-1.285), that tells us that Focus decreases when Bread increases. If the coefficient had been positive, then that would indicate increasing amounts of Bread correlate with increasing amounts of Focus. In regressions where you test a treatment that positively impacts focus, such as a supplement, you will notice a positive coefficient value for that supplement.

Example #6
A Simple Analysis of Medication and Eggs for Breakfast

Many people claim that eating a high protein breakfast, particularly eggs, significantly increases the efficacy of prescription stimulant medication. In this example, I demonstrate a simple analysis that determines whether this is true in a given situation.

Unlike the previous example, there is no need to deal with multiple time periods when you are simply testing the impact of a breakfast food on medication efficacy. In fact, we only need two columns of data, as shown in Figure 4.25.

Figure 4.25

Focus with medication	Eggs at breakfast
4	0
10	2
9	2
5	0
6	0
8	1
7	1
9	2
6	0
9	2
8	2
5	0

In this table, we have only one independent variable and the dependent variable. The dependent variable is simply a Focus score, with the added condition that it is an evaluation of focus while taking medication. This format of data can easily be created using information from your log, simply by isolating focus scores when a constant dose of medication has been consumed. Next, our independent variable is just the number of eggs consumed at breakfast. Our regression of the data follows.

Figure 4.26

Regression Statistics	
R Square	0.8664
Adjusted R Square	0.85304

ANOVA	
	Significance F
Regression	1.11131E-05

	Coefficients	P-value
Eggs at breakfast	1.9	1.11131E-05

Our regression results strongly indicate a positive relationship between focus while on medication and consuming eggs at breakfast. The R Square value indicates that egg consumption at breakfast explains 86 percent of the variation in focus while taking medication. Significance F and P-values are incredibly small, lending additional support to our assumption.

Finally, the coefficient value is positive, which tells us that the relationship between Eggs and Focus while on medication is positive. In summary, this sample analysis tells us that more eggs equal more focus when taking medication.

Example #7
Using Charts to Examine Long Term Improvement

In some instances, it is helpful to analyze data by using a chart instead of regression analysis. This is because some forms of improvement take time. For instance, prescription Atomoxetine medications do not work immediately the way stimulant medications do and may take a few weeks before any effects are realized. Furthermore, supplements like Ginkgo Biloba have been reported to take time before working. In these cases, we can evaluate improvement graphically, at least in the beginning.

Figure 4.27

Date	Focus	Date	Focus
1-Apr	4	16-Apr	6
2-Apr	3	17-Apr	5
3-Apr	4	18-Apr	6
4-Apr	4	19-Apr	7
5-Apr	3	20-Apr	6
6-Apr	4	21-Apr	7
7-Apr	3	22-Apr	8
8-Apr	3	23-Apr	7
9-Apr	4	24-Apr	6
10-Apr	5	25-Apr	8
11-Apr	4	26-Apr	7
12-Apr	4	27-Apr	9
13-Apr	5	28-Apr	8
14-Apr	5	29-Apr	8
15-Apr	4	30-Apr	9

Figure 4.28

Focus

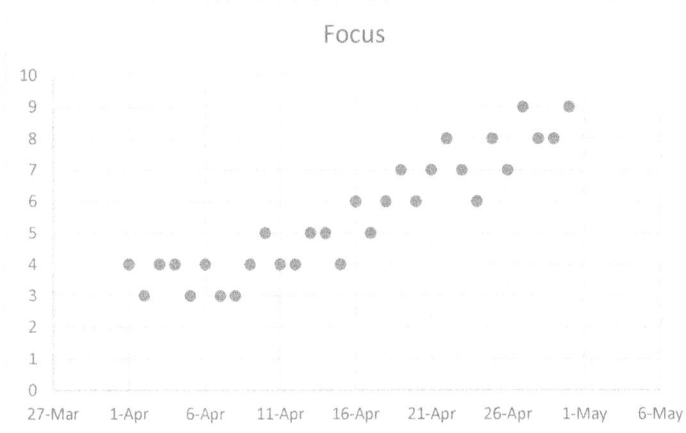

When a graph is intended to reveal the nature of a relationship between two variables, it is best to use a scatter plot as we have done thus far. In this example, a scatter plot works just fine to illustrate a focus trend with time. However, it is also acceptable to use a line graph in cases where we are graphing a single variable over time. The next page illustrates a line graph of the data.

Figure 4.29

Focus

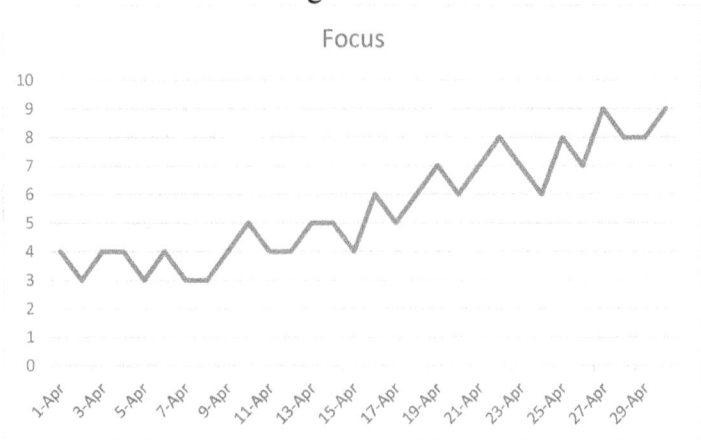

Both of these charts demonstrate that focus has increased during the month of April. Let's assume that the data represents a gradual increase in focus due to a supplement such as Ginkgo Biloba that needs to build up in the body. Using regression analysis to study the effect of the supplement on focus can cloud the results, so to speak. This is due to the fact that if the supplement takes time to work, our early evaluations of focus are not accurate representations of its effect. On April 30th we see that focus is all the way up to nine, but if we had included the beginning scores of three and four in the regression, that data would have ruined the credibility of the supplement in a regression.

For example, let's use the Focus scores from the month of April and run a regression of those scores with the inclusion of a Supplement independent variable. For the sake of comparison, in this example let's say that we did not take a supplement during the first two days of the month. We will fill the rest of the Supplement column with the number one to indicate that we did take the supplement during the remainder of the month, as sampled below.

Figure 4.30

Focus	Supplement
4	0
3	0
4	1
4	1
3	1

Figure 4.31 below shows the regression results.

Figure 4.31

Regression Statistics	
R Square	0.085626841
Adjusted R Square	0.052970657

ANOVA	
	Significance F
Regression	0.116597197

	P-value
Supplement	0.116597197

The regression results indicate that the supplement really has nothing to do with focus. However, this is simply because we did not account for the fact that the supplement needs time to begin working. If we run the regression again using only the first two days (our baseline for focus without the supplement) and the last two days (our values for focus during the full effect of the supplement), our results will be more accurate. The revised regression follows.

Figure 4.32

Regression Statistics	
R Square	0.961538462
Adjusted R Square	0.942307692
ANOVA	
	Significance F
Regression	0.019419324
	P-value
Supplement	0.019419324

The revised regression clearly shows that the supplement does indeed influence focus. Thus, we have demonstrated the problem with running a regression when the influence of a variable is changing over time.

Does this mean that we can never conduct a regression analysis using data on medications/supplements that take time to work? No. It simply means that if we want to conduct a regression on data that may be changing, we need to be careful **not to include any data while the**

change is occurring. What I mean by this is that when collecting data for use in a regression analysis, only include data for a medication/supplement you are taking when it is having its full effect. If it takes the supplement a month to start working, only include daily focus data *after* you have taken the supplement continuously for at least a month. By the same token, you should only record data representing days when it is not being taken if the supplement is not exerting any influence. This could include data based on *before* the supplement is taken, or well after it has left the body following discontinuation.

Thankfully, most of the time, we do not have to deal with independent variables that take an extended period of time to affect a dependent variable. In most cases, a straightforward analysis using regression is all that is necessary. However, it is important to be aware of this reality given the profound impact it can have on your analysis. A good example of this would be increasing vitamin intake due to deficiencies, as it can take a while for many nutrients to build up in the body. No matter what avenue of treatment you pursue, it is helpful to periodically graph out focus/hyperactivity control over time to evaluate how the overall treatment may be fluctuating in the long run.

Example #8
Testing for Tolerance and Applying Adjustments

Tolerance is a term we use to describe the phenomenon whereby a fixed dose of medication yields decreasing benefit over time. The effect may also occur when using certain herbal supplements. This occurrence is common among many different classes of medication and, unfortunately, it is very frequently observed in the treatment of ADHD with stimulants. This presents a challenge because if the effects of medications or supplements are changing, this will decrease the accuracy of a regression analysis. Therefore, it is important to recognize and compensate for tolerance when it occurs.

Maintaining a graph that visually illustrates long-term treatment success is the first step toward identifying tolerance. This would include a restricted graph that only shows focus/hyperactivity on days when you take a medication or supplement. If you notice that your graph has drastically decreased with time, tolerance may be the culprit.

If you or your child take stimulant medications but also skip medication on certain days, you can create scatter plots that will reveal whether or not the benefit from the medication decreases as it is taken longer continuously. Say, for example, that you take a stimulant medication Monday through Friday but do not take any on the weekend. You can organize this information, extracted

from a large set of journal entries, as shown in Figure
4.33.

Figure 4.33

Days Since Break	Focus	Stimulant (mg)
1	9	20
2	8	20
3	8	20
4	7	20
5	5	20
1	10	20
2	9	20
3	8	20
4	7	20
5	6	20
1	9	20
2	9	20
3	8	20
4	7	20
5	7	20

In this data set, we have arranged Focus and Stimulant
information from various journal entries according to
how long it has been since the last medication break. In
the context of our medication on weekdays example,
Day 1 represents Mondays, 2 represents Tuesdays and so
forth. The Stimulant (mg) column is only included as a
reference, and should not be included in the plot.

Creating a scatter plot of the previous information (stimulant dose excluded) yields the following.

Figure 4.34

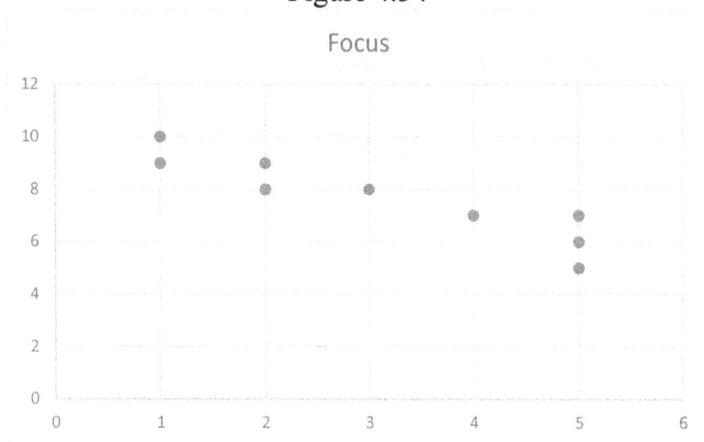

Focus

This is the default result when we create a scatter plot of the information. It is sufficient for identifying the day-to-day trend, but I will make some adjustments to ensure clarity. The reformatted scatter plot is on the next page.

Figure 4.35

Tolerance Identification Plot

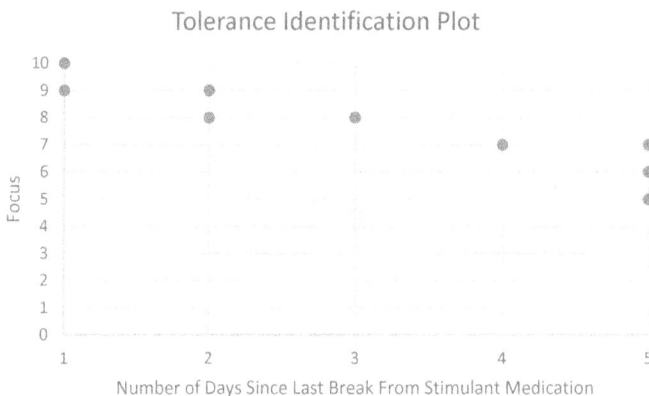

The plot shows that as you take the medication continuously over the course of five days, the benefit from the medication slowly decreases. Thus, it is clear that tolerance develops rather quickly, showing a decrease in benefit after only a few days of treatment.

Since we measure the data in a numerical format, you could also run a regression to test whether focus changes as the number of days of medication increases. Using Focus as the dependent variable and the number of days since the break as the independent variable, the results are as follows.

Figure 4.36

Regression Statistics		
R Square	0.853825137	
Adjusted R Square	0.842580916	
ANOVA		
	Significance F	
Regression	8.66508E-07	
	Coefficients	P-value
Days Since Break	-0.833333333	8.66508E-07

The regression confirms a relationship between focus while taking medication, and the number of days since the last break. Examining the negative coefficient tells us that as the number of days since a break increases, focus decreases.

However, this only looks at the first couple of days of medication use in an off/on scenario, and the treatment plan arranged with your health care provider may be very different. In many cases, providers prescribe stimulants at a low starting dose and then adjust to higher doses once tolerance begins to occur. This aims to achieve a steady level of long-term benefit, and further tolerance may not become a problem for weeks, months, or even years.

Because treatment plans differ so much, you may need to be a little bit creative when it comes to creating charts that will expose any tolerance effects. It is very important to remember, though, that we cannot allow inconsistencies to spoil our data. For instance, if you are charting focus levels while taking medication after breaks, it is sloppy technique to chart medication efficacy after breaks significantly different in duration. If you take medication after only one day off medication, focus on that day may be much different compared to what it would be after an entire week off medication. Tolerance to stimulant medication tends to decrease over time when breaks are taken, so it is important to maintain consistency if you want your analysis to be accurate and free of confusion.

This brings us to the challenge of compensating for tolerance in regressions and our overall analysis. In most cases when we use regression analysis, more data is better. The more often we observe something, the better we can understand its behavior, and so we aim to collect as much data as possible. Unfortunately, when tolerance is a factor, this limits our abilities to a certain extent. If we want to analyze the effect of a medication or supplement when it is working the way we expect it to consistently work, then we need to eliminate data from our analysis that does not represent the usual function of that substance. Observe the following graph that plots focus over the course of a month of medication use.

Figure 4.37

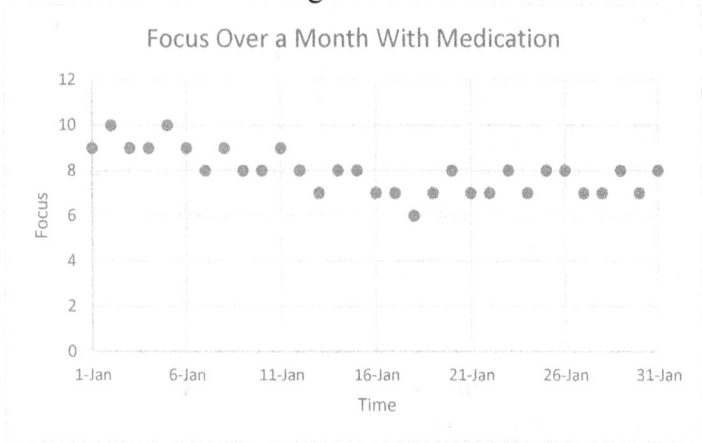

Focus Over a Month With Medication

In this graph, we notice that when medication usage commences at the beginning of the month, focus starts out pretty high. During the first six days, focus is assigned a score of nine or ten daily. As time goes on, we observe a minimal amount of increasing tolerance, and daily focus seems to settle at the seven to eight level. In order to analyze the benefit of medication properly, we need to omit the first week or so of data. Since the dose of medication is constant, if data is included that is not consistent with the long-term use of the medication, this can cloud our results.

Let's demonstrate the problem by including inconsistent information. On the next page is chart information from December when no medication was used.

Figure 4.38

Date	Focus	Medication (mg)
20-Dec	3	0
21-Dec	4	0
22-Dec	3	0
23-Dec	2	0
24-Dec	5	0
25-Dec	4	0
26-Dec	3	0
27-Dec	6	0
28-Dec	4	0
29-Dec	5	0
30-Dec	5	0
31-Dec	4	0

Using the December information as a baseline, let's compare two regressions: one that includes the December data, as well as the information from the entire month of January, and another that includes the data from December, but only the entries from January 12th onward.

First, we observe the results of the all-inclusive combined data.

Figure 4.39

Regression Statistics	
R Square	0.761908012
Adjusted R Square	0.75610089
ANOVA	
	Significance F
Regression	2.35566E-14
	P-value
Medication (mg)	2.35566E-14

Next, we see the results when we exclude the January data prior to the 12th.

Figure 4.40

Regression Statistics	
R Square	0.806511628
Adjusted R Square	0.800062016
ANOVA	
	Significance F
Regression	3.18477E-12
	P-value
Medication (mg)	3.18477E-12

Notice that in the revised regression, the R Square is larger, and the Significance F and P-value are slightly larger as well. The R Square is larger because our Focus values during the days with medication better reflect the true effects of the medication, and therefore the model can do a better job of explaining how medication impacts the variation of focus. The P-value and Significance F value became slightly larger because the original inclusion of the first couple of days in January gave the medication more credibility than it actually has in the long-run in terms of impacting focus. However, it would not be appropriate to include the first few days with excellent focus in the analysis simply because it makes the medication appear to have greater significance. If, instead, we remove declining Focus values from the end of a long-term chart of data because tolerance effects began to occur, this increases the significance of the medication, and rightly so.

It is critical that we use good judgment while performing an analysis that involves tolerance. The technique you use will largely depend on your particular situation and the perspective from which you interpret the data. If you are analyzing focus when you take medication every day over the long term, it makes sense to exclude any data that does not represent the actual long-term effects.

If you or your child only take medication five days a week and experience a slight decrease in effectiveness each day, as shown in the first part of this example, then it might make sense to go ahead and include logs for every day in your regression data. Although the data lacks perfect consistency, including all of it will give you results that represent the overall benefit of the medication. If the declining effect of medication is the same from week to week, you could select one specific day per week to include in your data, achieving significant consistency. Unfortunately, doing so would require several months to accumulate enough data for an accurate analysis. After keeping a journal for several months, you can always go back and put together the data that will yield results that are more meaningful.

Chapter 4 – Appendix A
Converting Data for Positive/Negative Relationship Analysis

In the first example of Chapter 4, we dealt with the issue of positive and negative relationships, and formatting our data entries accordingly. In Appendix A, we will investigate this a little further by demonstrating a shortcut in Excel that can modify the nature of what our entries represent.

In Example #1, we started our work with the data set in Figure 4.1, as shown below.

Figure 4.1

Date	Hyperactivity	Supplement 1 (mg)
1-Jan	8	0
2-Jan	7	0
3-Jan	4	500
4-Jan	6	0
5-Jan	2	750
6-Jan	6	0
7-Jan	7	0
8-Jan	3	500
9-Jan	3	500
10-Jan	5	500
11-Jan	5	0
12-Jan	1	750

The example used Hyperactivity as the dependent variable, and Supplement 1 as the independent variable. You'll notice that if the supplement is beneficial (which it is), we expect to see hyperactivity *decrease* when the supplement increases. In statistics, this constitutes a negative relationship, since one variable decreases when the other increases. This is the opposite of an analysis using Focus as the dependent variable since we expect to see focus *increase* when a medication, supplement or other factor confers benefit.

For some, it may be easier to think about things in terms of a positive relationship where variables increase or decrease together. If your journal data contains a column that ranks hyperactivity, you can easily convert those numbers into a corresponding Hyperactivity Management Score, which has a positive relationship with most independent variables. You can do this by completing the following steps.

1. In the first row of an empty column, type "Hyperactivity Management Score" or something similar to label the column.

2. In the second row of the column, type the appropriate variation of this equation: "=10-A2" where A2 represents the first box containing your hyperactivity data. Each box in an Excel worksheet has a unique letter/number identifier, allowing you to use the column letters and row numbers surrounding the data to specify exact boxes. If the hyperactivity information in your worksheet is in column N, and the first number begins in

row three, then you would modify the above equation to the following: "=10-N3" which corresponds to the appropriate box. Do not include quotation marks. Press "ENTER" when finished typing the equation. After you have entered the equation, the box should display the calculated number.

3. Assuming that the equation has been entered correctly, you can now command Excel to run the same calculation–subtracting the corresponding hyperactivity values from ten–down the rest of the column automatically. We do this by selecting the box we entered the first equation into. Click inside the box once so that a thick green border appears around the box. Next, move your mouse pointer to the bottom right hand corner of the box, where a black cross symbol will appear. Click and hold the left mouse button down while you drag the cursor down the column, until you reach a point with sufficient space in the column to fit the calculated information. Release the mouse. Excel should have filled the column with numbers calculated using the numbers in the Hyperactivity column.

Following this procedure for the data in Example #1 yields the following column of data.

Figure 4A.1

Hyperactivity Management Score
2
3
6
4
8
4
3
7
7
5
5
9

When entering an equation, the equals sign "=" tells Excel that you are typing an equation into the box and that Excel should run the calculation when you finish. In this example, we are subtracting the Hyperactivity score from 10 in order to create a Hyperactivity Management Score, which simply represents how well hyperactivity has been managed as opposed to representing the severity of hyperactivity. Since we scored hyperactivity on a scale of 0 to 10, it makes sense that subtracting these scores from ten would represent a score of how well hyperactivity was controlled. Looking over the data, we notice that the first day we scored hyperactivity as 8, and the corresponding value for hyperactivity management is 2. On the last day, we scored hyperactivity as only 1, rendering a Hyperactivity

Management Score of 9. Thus, we have converted the data in a way that allows us to explain our dependent variable as positively related to most independent variables.

Chapter 4 – Appendix B
A Bonus Analysis Example

In Appendix B, we will go through a larger example that demonstrates some of the essential skills learned in this book. Our journal data takes up the next two pages.

Figure 4B.1

Date	Focus	Hyperactivity	Med (mg)	Supp 1 (mg)	Supp 2	Supp 3 (mg)	Sleep	Egg B-Fast
1-Jan	4	7	0	0	0	0	7	0
2-Jan	5	7	0	0	1	0	8	1
3-Jan	9	3	30	10	1	50	8.5	1
4-Jan	8	3	30	10	1	50	8.5	0
5-Jan	6	5	30	10	0	0	8.5	0
6-Jan	6	5	0	0	0	0	9	1
7-Jan	6	2	0	0	1	50	8	1
8-Jan	8	8	30	10	0	0	8.5	0
9-Jan	3	2	0	0	0	0	2	1
10-Jan	7	4	30	10	1	50	7	0
11-Jan	10	2	30	10	1	50	9	1
12-Jan	6	3	30	0	1	50	8.5	0
13-Jan	5	4	0	0	0	50	8	1
14-Jan	4	8	0	0	1	0	8.5	1
15-Jan	7	5	30	10	0	0	8	0

Date								
16-Jan	10	4	30	10	1	0	8	1
17-Jan	2	8	0	0	1	0	8.5	1
18-Jan	5	6	0	10	0	0	8	1
19-Jan	8	1	30	0	0	50	8	0
20-Jan	4	2	0	0	1	50	8.5	1
21-Jan	9	4	30	10	1	50	8	1
22-Jan	3	3	0	0	0	50	8.5	1
23-Jan	8	2	30	10	1	50	9	1
24-Jan	7	5	30	0	1	0	8	0
25-Jan	4	9	0	0	0	0	7.5	1
26-Jan	3	1	0	0	1	50	8.5	1
27-Jan	8	2	30	10	0	50	8	0
28-Jan	9	2	30	10	0	50	8	1
29-Jan	7	5	30	0	1	0	9	0
30-Jan	8	3	30	0	0	50	8.5	1
31-Jan	6	7	0	10	1	0	7.5	0

As you can see, our journal includes two dependent variables–Focus and Hyperactivity. Because regression only works with one dependent variable, we will have to analyze focus and hyperactivity separately. Remember not to accidentally include one of your dependent variables as an independent variable in the regression for another dependent variable or your results will be incorrect.

Beginning with focus, we conduct a multiple regression using Focus as the dependent variable, and all variables shown to the right of Hyperactivity as independent variables.

Figure 4B.2

Regression Statistics	
R Square	0.792100494
Adjusted R Square	0.740125617

ANOVA	
	Significance F
Regression	3.87571E-07

	P-value
Med (mg)	1.1268E-05
Supp 1 (mg)	0.032283049
Supp 2	0.941891429
Supp 3 (mg)	0.904392657
Sleep	0.468772295
Egg B-Fast	0.087119505

We see that Supplements 2 and 3 have extremely high P-values, so we remove them and run the regression again.

Figure 4B.3

Regression Statistics	
R Square	0.791913561
Adjusted R Square	0.759900263
ANOVA	
	Significance F
Regression	1.549E-08
	P-value
Med (mg)	1.3594E-06
Supp 1 (mg)	0.025877986
Sleep	0.415951442
Egg B-Fast	0.052896513

Removing the insignificant supplements has not improved the Sleep variable by much, which is still much greater than the P-value cutoff of 0.05. Even though sleep may have the ability to impact focus, given the fact that sleep is relatively consistent from day to day, the model may not pick up on its significance. Since it does not meet our standards, we remove the Sleep variable and run the regression again.

Figure 4B.4

Regression Statistics	
R Square	0.78644434
Adjusted R Square	0.762715933

ANOVA	
	Significance F
Regression	3.38566E-09

	P-value
Med (mg)	3.47455E-07
Supp 1 (mg)	0.026293276
Egg B-Fast	0.040535463

Now that we have revised our multiple regression twice, this third regression includes three independent variables, all of which are below the P-value cutoff. However, it is possible that the Egg Breakfast variable does not influence focus on its own but rather makes the medication work better than it otherwise would. We can test this by using some of the techniques learned in Chapter 4. Let's start by isolating the way Focus changes when Medication and Supplement 1 are not taken. Since the Medication and Supplement 1 are both significant, we need to make sure that both remain fixed when studying Egg Breakfasts and Focus so that our results are accurate. Pulling from our original journal entries, we find twelve days when neither the Medication nor Supplement 1 were taken.

Figure 4B.5

Focus	Med (mg)	Supp 1 (mg)	Egg B-Fast
4	0	0	0
5	0	0	1
6	0	0	1
6	0	0	1
3	0	0	1
5	0	0	1
4	0	0	1
2	0	0	1
4	0	0	1
3	0	0	1
4	0	0	1
3	0	0	1

It would be better if we had more information about focus on days when no egg breakfast was consumed. You'll notice that we only have one entry with no egg breakfast. This data is sufficient for our example, but in real life it would be good to try skipping the Medication, Supplement 1 and an Egg Breakfast for a few more days to get a better sample. We reformat this information into the following.

Figure 4B.6

Focus (No Medication or Supplement 1)	Egg B-Fast
4	0
5	1
6	1
6	1
3	1
5	1
4	1
2	1
4	1
3	1
4	1
3	1

Running a regression of the data gives the following result.

Figure 4B.7

Regression Statistics	
R Square	0.000447828
Adjusted R Square	-0.099507389
ANOVA	
	Significance F
Regression	0.947952853
	P-value
Egg B-Fast	0.947952853

Viewing these regression results, it is apparent that an egg breakfast does nothing by itself to promote focus. Therefore, its success in the original model must be due to a relationship with one or more of the independent variables promoting focus. We can test this by isolating Egg Breakfast information when fixed amounts of Medication and Supplement 1 are consumed.

Figure 4B.8

Focus	Med (mg)	Supp 1 (mg)	Egg B-Fast
9	30	10	1
8	30	10	0
6	30	10	0
8	30	10	0
7	30	10	0
10	30	10	1
7	30	10	0
10	30	10	1
9	30	10	1
8	30	10	1
8	30	10	0
9	30	10	1

We reformat this information as follows.

Figure 4B.9

Focus (Med & Supp 1 taken)	Egg B-Fast
9	1
8	0
6	0
8	0
7	0
10	1
7	0
10	1
9	1
8	1
8	0
9	1

Running a regression gives us the following.

Figure 4B.10

Regression Statistics	
R Square	0.620512821
Adjusted R Square	0.582564103
ANOVA	
	Significance F
Regression	0.002347294
	P-value
Egg B-Fast	0.002347294

The second regression testing the impact of an egg breakfast reveals that eggs do in fact have an influence on how well the medication and supplement improve focus. The R Square is only 0.62, indicating that whether or not an egg breakfast is consumed only accounts for 62 percent of the variation in Focus that occurs when we take both the medication and supplement. However, the Significance F and P-value tell us that the breakfast is significant when combined with the medication and supplement. Based on these findings, we can deduce that although an egg breakfast does not improve focus on its own, it is advisable to eat an egg breakfast on days you take the medication and supplement.

Moving on now to hyperactivity, we run the regression with Hyperactivity as the dependent variable along with all of the original independent variables.

Figure 4B.11

Regression Statistics	
R Square	0.694623376
Adjusted R Square	0.61827922

ANOVA

	Significance F
Regression	3.08927E-05

	P-value
Med (mg)	0.099400674
Supp 1 (mg)	0.446578925
Supp 2	0.939000973
Supp 3 (mg)	4.29824E-06
Sleep	0.031187353
Egg B-Fast	0.472308592

Since Supplements 1 and 2, along with Egg Breakfast have high P-values, we run the regression again with those variables omitted.

Figure 4B.12

Regression Statistics	
R Square	0.681469313
Adjusted R Square	0.646077014
ANOVA	
	Significance F
Regression	7.00657E-07
	P-value
Med (mg)	0.157307129
Supp 3 (mg)	2.27345E-07
Sleep	0.023544172

In the revised regression, Medication still has not come down to an acceptable P-value, so we remove it from the model.

Figure 4B.13

Regression Statistics		
R Square	0.6565075	
Adjusted R Square	0.631972322	
ANOVA		
	Significance F	
Regression	3.18304E-07	
	Coefficients	P-value
Supp 3 (mg)	-0.074994782	6E-08
Sleep	0.448193005	0.043977

Our final regression results indicate that Supplement 3 and Sleep both influence Hyperactivity, but they only explain 63 percent of the variation in hyperactive behavior. This suggests that there are other factors, not included in our analysis, which may have a significant impact on hyperactive behavior. Interestingly, the Sleep coefficient is positive, which tells us that as sleep increases, so does hyperactivity. One explanation for this could be that as sleep decreases, the person is less likely to have the energy to behave hyperactively.

Conclusion

Thank you for taking the time to read this book. I hope that this information enables you to successfully improve your quality of life or that of a loved one. I enjoy receiving feedback from readers, so please contact me if you have any comments or suggestions on improving this book.

www.AustinTallman.com

References

[1] Skokauskas, N., McNicholas, F., Masaud, T., & Frodl, T. (2011). Complementary Medicine for Children and Young People Who Have Attention Deficit Hyperactivity Disorder. Current Opinion in Psychiatry, Retrieved from http://www.medscape.com/viewarticle/744677

[2] Mousain-Bosc, M., Roche, M., Polge, A., Pradal-Prat, D., Rapin, J., Bali, JP. (2006). Improvement of neurobehavioral disorders in children supplemented with magnesium-vitamin B6. Magnesium Research, Retrieved from http://www.jle.com/en/revues/bio_rech/mrh/e-docs/00/04/18/F1/article.phtml

[3] Konofal, E., Lecendreux, M., Arnulf, I., Mouren, M. (2004). Iron Deficiency in Children With Attention-Deficit/Hyperactivity Disorder. Archives of Pediatrics and Adolescent Medicine, Retrieved from http://archpedi.jamanetwork.com/article.aspx?articleid=485884

[4] Kemper, K. (2007). Lifestyle and Complementary Therapies for ADHD. Retrieved from http://www.medscape.org/viewarticle/554850_4

[5] Fehske, C., Leuner, K., Müller, W.E. (2009). Ginkgo biloba extract (EGb761®) influences monoaminergic neurotransmission via inhibition of NE uptake, but not MAO activity after chronic treatment, Pharmacological Research, 60(1), 68-73. Retrieved from http://www.ncbi.nlm.nih.gov/pubmed/19427589/?

[6] Lyon, M. R., Cline, J. C., Totosy de Zepetnek, J., Shan, J. J., Pang, P., & Benishin, C. (2001). Effect of the herbal extract combination Panax quinquefolium and Ginkgo biloba on attention-deficit hyperactivity disorder: a pilot study. Journal of Psychiatry and Neuroscience, Retrieved from http://www.ncbi.nlm.nih.gov/pmc/articles/PMC1408291/